CAREERS IN
RADIOLOGIC TECHNOLOGY

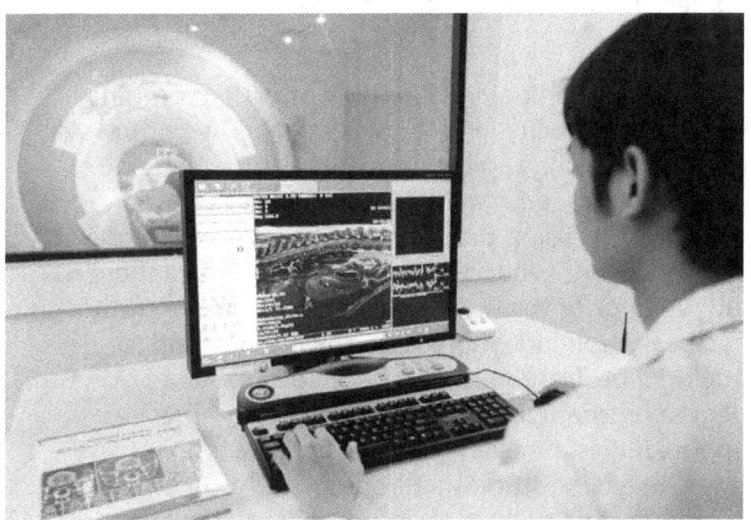

RADIOLOGIC TECHNOLOGISTS ARE THE HEALTHCARE professionals who perform medical imaging examinations used for diagnosing illness or injury. They use a variety of equipment that utilizes radiation to create the images, such as X-ray, magnetic resonance imaging (MRI), and computed tomography (CT). Some are also trained to administer radiation therapy treatments to cancer patients.

Radiologic technologists are often known by the type of technology they handle or the particular examination technique they perform. For example, there are MRI techs, CT techs, and X-ray techs as well as mammographers, sonographers, and nuclear medicine technologists.

Most radiologic technologists work in hospitals, but they are needed in every healthcare setting including doctors' offices, outpatient clinics, diagnostic and research laboratories, and independent diagnostic imaging centers. There are even traveling radiologic technologists who bring their well-equipped vans to patients in their homes, assisted living facilities, senior communities, and hospices.

A career in radiologic technology offers a promising future, job stability, and a good salary. The number of jobs is increasing rapidly because of the expanding population of aging adults – the primary users of diagnostic imaging procedures. That makes it a good choice for individuals who want to make sure there is a job waiting for them when they have completed the necessary training. There is a growing demand for qualified professionals who have completed a two-year degree program in radiologic technology. The opportunities are even greater for those who pursue more advanced studies and obtain certification in specializations such as radiation therapy or vascular interventional technology.

Salaries for radiologic technologists are very competitive with other healthcare professionals with similar educational backgrounds. The median annual income for a generalist is $60,000, and with the right combination of location and experience, it is possible to reach $85,000. Those who obtain the extra training needed for certification in other modalities can experience a boost in income. An MRI tech, for example, earns on average 25 percent more than a generalist.

Radiologic technologists do not have to worry about being laid off or getting bored. This is a stable career that offers many options. You could use your skills to work in pediatric care or orthopedics. You could teach or manage an entire radiology department. You could perform research that leads to breakthroughs in diagnostic imaging or radiation therapy. You could even get out of the hospital environment altogether and work with professional athletes. Once you have obtained the basic knowledge and skills, you can expand the boundaries of your career in any direction that interests you.

WHAT YOU CAN DO NOW

THIS IS A CAREER THAT REQUIRES some higher education. In addition to obtaining a high school diploma or its equivalent, it is important to prepare for college or technical school entrance requirements. In general, that includes four years of English, mathematics, and natural sciences. More specifically, schools with radiology programs like to see students who have completed courses in physics, chemistry, and biology. Candidates should also have a basic understanding of anatomy as well as computer skills.

To learn more about the profession and whether it is a good fit for you, talk to your school's guidance counselor about any resources that may be available. Ask for help in arranging a job shadow. You can arrange this for yourself, too. Simply call up local medical imaging services or the nearest hospital. Ask the radiology department head if you can come in to ask them some questions. Be sure to ask what they do and do not like about their job, and how they got to where they are today.

To get an even better idea of what the workplace experience is like, look for volunteer opportunities at your local hospital. Use this time to get acquainted with the work environment, talk to the practicing radiologic technologists, ask questions, and start deciding if you are a good fit for a job in the field of radiology. It is not always possible to land a volunteer position in the radiology department, but any position in healthcare will be a big plus on your résumé.

There are a number of professional associations for radiologic technologists. Look online to find one in your area that you can join and take advantage of their educational activities. Many have discounted student memberships and sponsor educational and networking events for students.

HISTORY OF THE CAREER

LIKE MANY GREAT DISCOVERIES, x-rays were discovered by accident. It happened in 1895 when German physics professor, Wilhelm Roentgen, was studying how electricity passed through cathode ray tubes. He noticed that the image left on a paper included details not found in an ordinary photograph. After some experimentation, he took the first successful x-ray. It was of his wife's hand, revealing images of her bones. What Roentgen discovered was a way to make transparent film images. He named it "x-ray" because of the mysterious nature of unknown rays that created the images. The implications of the technology were huge and Roentgen quickly became a celebrity. He won the first Nobel Prize in physics in 1901.

The medical community immediately recognized the value of x-ray technology in the diagnosis of broken bones, fractures, and various ailments. Less than a year after Roentgen took his first x-ray, crude x-ray machines were produced for use in the medical community. While the machines were being refined, physicians like Dr. Harvey Cushing sought new ways to use the technology in clinical settings. In 1902, Dr. Cushing began his groundbreaking work in surgery, including brain surgery, using x-rays to help locate and remove tumors.

In the early days of x-ray technology, physicians took the images themselves. The responsibilities were eventually shifted to staff members who were usually women already working in the doctors' offices as receptionists or nurses. The dangers of radiation exposure were unknown until 1915, and the machines were very unsafe. There were no safety devices, and people who worked with x-rays began dying at an alarmingly high rate.

Dr. Marie Curie is credited with discovering the radioactive metals, radium and polonium. Curie's work had a profound influence within the field of medicine. Among many things, Curie found that the harmful properties of x-rays were able to kill tumors. During World War I, she also designed radiology cars that brought x-ray machines to hospitals that treated wounded soldiers. It is estimated that she was responsible for making it possible to x-ray more than a million soldiers, many of whom were saved as a result. Ironically, Curie herself eventually died of leukemia, which was the result of repeated exposure to radioactive material. However, due to her work and discoveries in the field, safety advances were made that protect both patients and caregivers.

Ed Jerman, an American inventor, became fascinated with

x-ray technology. He was one of the first people to focus on the finer details of quality imaging. He was hired by Victor X-ray Corporation of General Electric's medical division, to train salespeople who were expected to demonstrate the company's x-ray machines. In 1916, Jerman started his own medical supply company and began training x-ray technicians in the safe and proper use of x-ray machines. Four years later, Jerman and a dozen x-ray technicians established the American Association of Radiological Technicians. Because of his early efforts to license personnel who took x-rays, he is often credited with creating the field of professional radiologic technology. His organization, which eventually became the American Society of Radiologic Technologists, worked tirelessly to persuade the federal government to establish standards for x-ray technicians that would ensure the protection of patients and technicians alike. This goal was finally accomplished with the signing of legislation in 1981.

Ultrasound

In the 1940s, several doctors from different countries studied the use of sonography within the medical field. Austrian physician, Karl Theodore, published the first paper on medical ultrasonic technology. He had been using transmission ultrasound to explore the brain. The 1942 paper reported on the results of his research. Dr. George Ludwig was the first American to use ultrasound for medical purposes. A professor of medicine and medical researcher, Dr. Ludwig initially used ultrasound to detect gallstones in the late 1940s. He wrote the first paper in the US on the use of ultrasound for diagnostic purposes.

The 1950s marked the beginning of a new technique that used ultrasound for noninvasive diagnostics within the field of cardiology. The technique was developed in Sweden by cardiologist, Inge Edler and physicist Carl

Hellmuth Hertz. It came about when Edler asked Hertz about the possibilities of using radar to look inside the human body. Hertz doubted radar would work, and suggested the use of ultrasonic sound instead. Hertz had used the technology in other applications, but not in the medical field. Together, the men figured out how to use it to accurately measure heart and brain activity. It was a landmark discovery that came to be known as echocardiography.

MRI Technology

The first full body MRI (Magnetic Resonance Imaging) scanner was built in the 1970s by a team led by Scottish professor John Mallard. It was first used in an actual clinical setting in 1980 to obtain an image of a patient's internal tissues. The scan correctly identified a primary tumor in the patient's chest, an abnormal liver, and secondary cancer in bones. A year later, researchers in California published *Nuclear Magnetic Resonance Imaging in Medicine.* The book was considered the definitive introductory textbook to the subject.

The first MRI exam took almost five hours to produce just one image. Today there are thousands of MRI scanners throughout the country with images being produced in minutes as opposed to hours.

CAT Scans

A CT (computerized tomography) or CAT scan (computerized axial tomography) uses a computer to retrieve data from several x-ray images to generate cross-sectional and/or three-dimensional views of the internal organs and structures of the body. The scans are generally used to define normal and abnormal structures in the body. They can also assist in medical procedures by helping to accurately guide the placement of instruments.

The original CT systems were intended for head imaging

only, but whole body systems with larger openings became available in 1976. Since then the technology has developed rapidly and continues to become more patient friendly and faster. The first CT took hours to acquire raw data, and took days to reconstruct a single image from that raw data. Today, multi-slice CT systems can collect up to four slices of data in about 350 milliseconds, and reconstruct an image from millions of data points in less than a second. Equally important for patients, researchers have also developed systems that produce excellent quality images at the lowest possible x-ray dose.

WHERE YOU WILL WORK

MOST RADIOLOGIC TECHNOLOGISTS WORK in general or surgical hospitals, the number one place of employment for these careerists. Of the 215,000 technicians working in the US today, approximately 130,000 work in local, state, or private hospitals. Most are assigned to critical areas like trauma, surgery, and angiography. Others work in the imaging department and may spend all their time in the CT or MRI rooms.

The next largest group of radiologic technicians, about one in five, work in doctors' offices or clinics. In the past, physicians were reluctant to invest in the expense of imaging equipment. They instead sent their patients to the nearest hospital with imaging orders. Today, imaging has become so vital to accurate and timely diagnostics that most doctors are now able to offer at least some medical radiological services in-house. Medical diagnostic laboratories and outpatient care centers are also major employers of radiologic technicians.

A fast-growing type of employer is the mobile imaging service. Medical equipment manufacturers have figured out how to shrink the size of X-ray, MRI, PET/CT, and CT machines. At first, that meant hospitalized patients did not need to be wheeled down to the imaging department for x-rays. Instead, the mobile x-ray operator would come to the patient's room and take images bedside. The service has expanded greatly, and mobile techs can now provide hospital-quality imaging services to homebound and non-ambulatory patients. This means that techs can work in many more environments, such as private residences, assisted living facilities, nursing homes, senior communities, sporting events, specialty clinics and treatment centers, and correctional institutions. In addition, they may work for home-care or hospice agencies, or corporate employers that provide on-site chest exams to staff.

Radiologic technologists can be found working in every state, in both cities and urban areas. Among the states, California and Texas offer the most jobs for this profession. Opportunities are especially abundant in the cities of New York, Los Angeles, and Chicago.

Work Schedules

Most radiologic technologists work full time, 40 hours a week. In hospitals, which are naturally much busier than most outpatient settings, positions often require evenings or weekend shifts. Because imaging is often needed in emergencies, those assigned to trauma units or emergency rooms may need to be on call or on duty overnight when needed.

Because there is such a high demand for trained personnel, opportunities for part-time, temporary, or shift work are also available. Sometimes technologists work part time for more than one hospital or clinic. This provides good flexibility, which is attractive to individuals who are raising families or who are pursuing additional education.

THE WORK YOU WILL DO

A RADIOLOGIC TECHNOLOGIST IS A CRITICAL MEMBER of the healthcare team. These professionals are trained to use a variety of sophisticated imaging equipment to examine the internal properties of the human body. They work closely with physicians who will use the images to diagnose a disease or injury, treat medical conditions that would otherwise require surgery, or conduct research. It is important that the images be clear and accurate in order for the radiologist to interpret them correctly.

The specific tasks of any particular radiologic technologist will depend on the type of equipment used, the purpose of the scan, and the patient's particular issues. The general routine is the same for all technologists. It starts with preparing the patient by describing what will happen during each step of the process. Occasionally, patients are anxious or stressed, and the technologist needs to patiently calm their fears. Patients are instructed to remove any clothing or jewelry that could interfere with the imaging process.

The technologist positions the patient carefully to ensure that the target area will be clearly captured on the image. When appropriate, parts of the body not being filmed are shielded to protect the patient from overexposure. In some cases, the technologist needs to inject the patient with a contrast agent such as barium or iodine to guarantee a high-quality image. The equipment is then focused and adjusted as necessary before taking the actual images. The technologist will review the results with the supervising radiologist and take additional views when necessary.

Imaging Types

Most technologists start out practicing general radiography. After a couple of years, they tend to gravitate toward a particular type of imaging equipment, technique, or treatment method. The most common kinds of equipment are X-rays, magnetic resonance imaging (MRI) scanners, and computerized tomographic (CT) scans.

X-ray is a type of radiation that can be used to produce black and white images of the human body. The images may be captured on film and/or computer. Most people think machines are only used to detect broken bones. It is more likely that the X-ray technologist will be asked to examine the chest and look for signs of pneumonia. The technologist can also use the equipment to look for foreign objects in the body and reveal dislocation between bone and soft tissue. X-ray technology is a common starting point in a radiologic technologist's career because it requires the least amount of education.

MRI technologists obtain additional training in how to operate MRI equipment. During a typical imaging procedure a patient is injected with a contrast dye that will make images glow on the scanner. During the MRI scan, the technologist applies a radio frequency pulse to the patient's body that knocks atoms out of alignment and creates a strong magnetic field. When the technologist turns the pulse off, the atoms give off signals as they return to their original position. A computer measures the signals and uses them to create detailed images.

CT technologists use a special rotating X-ray machine that can obtain "slices" of different levels within the body. A computer stacks and assembles the individual slices to create a three-dimensional image. CT scanners make it possible to see inside of organs, bones, blood vessels, and soft tissue – something X-rays cannot do. CT technologists typically work with one certain section of anatomy at a time, such as the abdomen, colon, or head.

Diagnostic Specializations

Radiologic technologists can also specialize in a particular type of diagnostic healthcare. One of the most common is mammography. Mammographers take X-rays of breast tissue to diagnose potential breast cancer. Special low-dose X-ray systems are used to produce these diagnostic images. Under the direction of a physician, the mammographer explains the procedure to the patient, positions and immobilizes the patient's breast in the X-ray unit, and observes the scanning process. There is a federal law known as the Mammography Quality Standards Act that requires radiologic technologists to meet strict educational and experience criteria in order to perform mammographic procedures.

Bone densitometry technologists use a different kind of X-ray machine designed to measure bone mineral density. Following a physician's prescription, the technologist typically targets a specific part of the patient's body, such as the hip, spine, wrist, or heel in order to estimate the risk of fracture. In some cases, the technologist will be tasked with calculating the total bone mineral content of the entire body. This is usually done when osteoporosis is suspected, or to monitor the rate of bone loss over a specific period of time.

Cardiac interventional and vascular interventional technologists use some of the most sophisticated imaging techniques such as biplane fluoroscopy and vascular ultrasound for both diagnostic and therapeutic purposes. They are responsible for administering ionizing radiation that can help guide catheters, vena cava filters, stents, or other medical tools through the body. The work of these highly skilled technologists can help doctors treat heart and vascular disease without the risks and long recovery of open surgery.

Nuclear medicine technologists use radioisotope equipment to obtain detailed information about a patient's organs, tissues, and/or bones. This requires subjecting patients to radiation, which means calculating dosages, preparing solutions, and administering tiny amounts of radioactive isotopes. A special camera is then used to detect the gamma rays emitted by the radiopharmaceutical solution. An image is created and information is recorded on a computer screen.

Sonographers conduct ultrasound examinations. Ultrasound equipment uses sound waves to obtain images of organs and tissues in the body. In ultrasound imaging, a transducer replaces the camera. The sonographer places the transducer on the area of the body being studied and applies an electric charge. That creates high-frequency sound waves that pass through the body and sends back echoes as it bounces off organs and tissues. Specialized computer software then converts the echoes into visual images that the sonographer is trained to read.

In every radiology department, there are radiologic technologists responsible for quality management. These professionals make sure the equipment and the processes used by staff are meeting high quality standards. They collect data and use information analysis tools and methods to monitor all activities in the department. Daily tasks typically include performing quality control tests on machinery, assessing film density, calibrating timers, evaluating team members' methodologies, and identifying production problems that may lead to inaccurate readings.

Radiation Oncology

While much of radiologic technology is about diagnosing health problems, it is also routinely used for treatment of many types of cancer. This type of treatment is known as radiation oncology. The radiation oncology team consists of a radiation oncologist, a medical physicist, and two kinds of radiological technologist: the medical dosimetrist and the radiation therapist.

The medical dosimetrist works closely with the medical physicist to determine how much radiation will be delivered to a tumor site. After a treatment plan is developed by the radiation oncologist, the medical dosimetrist uses their advanced knowledge of physics, anatomy, and radiobiology to calculate the optimal dosage for successful treatment. This is extremely exacting work because the dose must effectively kill the cancer cells in the targeted area while avoiding damage to nearby organs and healthy tissue surrounding the tumor.

Once the medical dosimetrist determines the dosage and target area, it is the radiation therapist who will actually administer treatment to the patient's body. These are highly-trained specialists who have received advanced education in patient anatomy, physics, radiation safety, and patient care. Unlike medical dosimetrists, they are in direct contact with patients. A typical treatment plan will last between four and seven weeks during which the radiation therapist will see a patient three to five times a week.

Other Team Members

There are two members of the radiologic team that perform similar tasks to those of the technologist: radiologic technicians and radiology assistants. The radiologic technician operates imaging equipment, positions patients for best results, and performs the tests that create digital images of the body for the purpose of diagnosing illness. Most technicians take X-rays, but they may also be trained to handle computed tomography (CT) scans or mammograms. So what is the difference between a technician and a technologist? It is mainly the level of training. A technician can get an entry-level job with as little as one year of training at a vocational-technology (Vo-Tech) school learning how to operate imaging equipment. Technologists need at least two years to qualify for certification and/or licensing.

There are also radiology assistants on the team. This is a fairly new occupation recognized by the American Registry of Radiologic Technologists. Radiology assistants are experienced, trained radiologic technologists who have completed the advanced study (four years minimum) required for licensing. They work directly under the supervision of a licensed radiologist (medical doctor) to manage patient care in the digital imaging environment. Like technologists, they perform radiologic procedures. Unlike technologists however, their job duties go a step farther to include taking a patient's medical history and doing a preliminary analysis of test results.

PERSONAL STORIES FROM PEOPLE IN THE CAREER

I Work at a Teaching Hospital

"I always wanted to be in the medical profession and started college with the intention of becoming a nurse. When I learned there was a very long waiting list to get into the nursing program, my guidance counselor suggested looking into the radiologic technology program. I wasn't sure I'd like it at first, but it turned out to be a great choice. I've been in this career for more than 25 years now and never regretted it for a moment. I spent most of my career working in different hospital departments, but the most satisfying work I've done is teaching future professionals.

I have noticed that too many students come unprepared for the course work in a radiologic technology program. It's important to do some homework before enrolling. You should know what the work involves and what technologists actually do each day. Get the college catalog while in high school and make sure you have the necessary prerequisites. Pay attention in algebra and English – they will be on your placement exams and your college instruction will build on your knowledge. Don't assume that because most radiologic technology programs are in community colleges that means it will be easy. The reality is that four years of information is stuffed into two years. There is nothing easy about that!

The best advice I can offer to new radiologic technologists is to branch out. Work in as many different environments as you can. Unless you explore the possibilities, you will never know how far you could go in your career. Also, be sure to get actively involved in professional organizations. It's the best way to find people who can connect you with wonderful opportunities that otherwise would not come your way."

I Work for an NFL Team

"Everyone loves to watch the rough and tumble game of football. But did you know that there are 30 medical personnel standing ready at every NFL game? There are three medical teams: home team, visiting team, and stadium team. As a member of the stadium team, I am responsible for both teams before, during, and after the game. I'm proud that I play a role in taking care of so many fine athletes.

When I started 15 years ago, there was only a tiny X-ray room and it was assumed most injuries were orthopedic. Now each stadium has a state-of-the-art trauma radiographic room with fluoroscopic imaging capabilities that allow me to send digital images directly to the trauma physicians on the sidelines. Our understanding of injuries has evolved to include chronic traumatic encephalopathy (CTE) and traumatic spine and brain injuries. I've been trained to look for subtle signs of injuries to the brain during the imaging process even when the player is in the X-ray room for a specific orthopedic injury. This has become a very important part of my job.

I've learned to pay attention to all sorts of details that

help me pinpoint what kind of imaging would help get an accurate diagnosis. From watching each individual player, I will notice if there is a change in personality or behavior that could indicate a concussion. There are also certain injuries that are common to players in certain positions, such as shoulder injuries in quarterbacks or knee injuries in defensive linemen. Watching for these potential 'positional injuries' helps me understand what a player needs at any given time. The lingo of professional football is another source of inside information that helps me know how to do my job. For example, a player might tell me he got 'chopped' and while a radiologic technologist in the local hospital wouldn't have any idea what that meant, I know the common injuries associated with that term. These are the details that can make the difference between a quick diagnosis and successful treatment, and long term health problems."

I Work With Cancer Patients

"I work in radiation therapy as a certified medical dosimetrist. I work behind the scenes to design a treatment plan and make calculations for the delivery of radiation based on the oncology physician's prescribed course of therapy. Each treatment plan is different because each patient is different. I need to consider the tumor pathology, tumor volume, the location in the body, and any tissue or organ near the tumor that will necessarily limit dosage. In short, it's my responsibility to make sure that the radiation will kill the cancer, but not harm the patient. I accomplish this with complex computer equipment and a whole lot of math.

My education included all kinds of science and anatomy courses related to cancer treatment and brachytherapy (internal radiation), but it was math that turned out to be the most important. In fact, my whole job is math related. Most of the time I can use specialized software to calculate optimum dosages based on size of the treatment field, type of energy to be used (photon, electron, or gamma ray), and type of structure that surrounds the tumor. Sometimes I also do manual calculations to determine precisely how long each treatment needs to continue to reach a certain depth.

This is a discipline that has been very rewarding. I'm a valued member of the radiation oncology team and what I do makes a difference in a patient's life. I wasn't sure where or how I wanted to apply my radiologic technology skills when I first started. After making the rounds of a few other modalities, I came across radiation oncology and immediately knew it was the career for me. I would advise all new radiologic technologists to do the same – try different things to find the right fit. And make sure you pay attention in math class!"

PERSONAL QUALIFICATIONS

RADIOLOGIC TECHNOLOGY IS CONSIDERED A HIGH-touch, high-tech field. Technical expertise is obviously needed, but an excellent bedside manner is equally important. Technologists may see patients only briefly, but in that short period of time they must use soft skills like effective communication, patience, and interpersonal skills. They work closely with patients who may be experiencing extreme pain. Some will be alone with no family support to ease their fears and stress. The technologist must be able to make patients comfortable, both emotionally and physically, in order to get usable images. It is not always easy to pinpoint the location and level of pain a patient is experiencing, especially in the emergency room, but it is an essential part of the job.

Successful radiologic technologists have an aptitude for science and technology that serves them well during training. After graduating, they must understand how to operate complex machinery. The imaging career is continually developing. For example, though most hospitals have 64 slice CT scanners, there are now 256 slice and 320 slice scanners available. Having a keen interest in new and advancing technologies will be helpful because the best way to succeed in this career is to keep current through workshops and seminars, reading professional journals, and pursuing continuing education opportunities.

A head for math is also an advantage since these technologists may need to calculate and mix the right doses of chemicals used in imaging procedures.

You might not think of this as a physically demanding profession but actually it does require some strength and stamina. Moving and positioning patients to get accurate images are an important part of the job. Some patients are going to be quite heavy and others are going to be unable to move themselves due to pain or possibly even being unconscious. For that reason, employers generally require technologists to be able to lift at least 50 pounds. Radiologic technologists who work in hospitals often work long shifts, which means they are on their feet for many hours. This could be quite tiring for someone who is not physically fit.

Radiologic technologists should be detail oriented. Doctors often give precise instructions that must be followed exactly to get the images needed for accurate diagnoses. Critical and creative thinking are also extremely important. Many new technologists assume that how they learned to do things in school is the only way. In fact, it is only a guideline. Each patient has different issues and the technologist must think outside the box when determining the best way to perform the examination on a patient.

ATTRACTIVE FEATURES

ACCORDING TO NUMEROUS SURVEYS of radiologic technologists, this is a great career choice for anyone who wants to do interesting and satisfying work. It is ranked high among the best jobs in healthcare for numerous reasons, including job stability, easy entry, good pay, flexibility, and a promising future.

Every individual who gets the requisite training can expect to find a job waiting. This is a fast growing field with immediate and sustainable demand for trained professionals in hospitals, clinics, and doctors' offices. Employment experts predict much faster job growth in this field than for all other occupations on average. That means job security is assured well into the foreseeable future.

Getting started is relatively quick and easy. A one-year certificate or a two year associate degree is all it takes to get started in most entry-level positions. There are also bachelor's and master's degree programs in radiology or applied health sciences available for those who intend to advance to the highest level in their profession. With additional education and a few years of work experience, a radiologic technologist can take advantage of excellent opportunities for advancement into specialized modalities or even into management.

The pay is very good, especially considering the relatively small investment in training. In fact, radiologic technologists enjoy one of the highest starting salaries of vocational careers. By taking advantage of continuing education opportunities, these professionals can get certified in specialty areas that pay at least 25 percent more than the generalists typically get. For example, a certified MRI technologist in a major city hospital can earn close to six figures. That is a good return for training for an extra one or two years.

One of the best features of this career is the variety of options. There is no reason to ever be bored! There are numerous specializations to choose from including ultrasound, MRI, CT, mammography, cancer, and trauma. There are also various medical settings to choose from. The majority of radiologic technologists work in hospitals, but there are many opportunities in outpatient centers, physicians' offices, and clinics. Even in the hospital environment, a tech can work throughout the facility rather than in just one spot. For those who prefer to move around, there are mobile imaging agencies that send technologists out in large well-equipped vans to service patients in their homes, assisted living facilities, corporate workplaces, and correctional facilities. There are also scheduling options. Most radiologic technologists work full time, but there are part-time and temporary opportunities for those who need some flexibility.

UNATTRACTIVE ASPECTS

RADIOLOGIC TECHNOLOGISTS REPORT VERY FEW or no downsides to their career choice. Most say their jobs turned out to be exactly what they expected and they are very satisfied with the work. Nonetheless, there are a few points to consider before forging ahead.

One of the attractive features of this career is the relatively short education requirements. Most healthcare careers take many years of intense education. Compare that to just two years to obtain a solid foundation on which to build your career. While that is a relatively short time, the training program will not be easy. Like most healthcare professions, required courses include difficult subjects like advanced anatomy, pathology, chemistry, and physiology. Add to that just about every radiologic procedure and theory there is, and you have a heavy load of homework, hours of reading outside class, lab work, and clinical projects. By the time you have graduated, it will be a relief to get to work.

As in many other healthcare professions, radiologic technologists may be exposed to infectious diseases. There are also risks associated with working with imaging equipment that uses radiation. These hazards are minimized by wearing protective lead vests or aprons. For some tests, such as ultrasounds, protective gloves are used. Badges that measure radiation levels are also worn in the radiation area. Detailed records are kept of each technologist's lifetime cumulative exposure to radiation.

There was a time when this field was considered a "lifestyle specialty" because the hours were regular and schedules were flexible. However, more and more hospitals are expanding their hours to accommodate heavier caseloads and accommodate patients who cannot get away from work during normal business hours. This has caused shifts to include evenings, weekends, and some holidays. Plus, some departments require technologists to be on call when they are not on site.

The work can be physically tiring. Technologists must be able to lift or turn heavy or disabled patients. Hiring requirements generally stipulate the ability to lift at least 50 pounds or more. Most of the time, radiologic technologists are on their feet, which can be very tiring when the shifts are long.

Most people go into healthcare professions because they want to help people. Radiologic technology is no exception. However, the level of patient contact in this work is minimal compared to some others like nursing or physical therapy. There is some patient contact during examinations and imaging procedures, but it is brief. Still, there is a sense of satisfaction in knowing diagnostic and interventional radiology greatly impacts patient care and outcomes.

EDUCATION AND TRAINING

THERE IS MORE THAN ONE WAY TO PREPARE for a career in radiologic technology. The most common is to enroll in a two-year associate degree program at a community college. Vo-tech schools often offer certificate programs that can be completed in less than 24 months. Some hospitals provide their own training programs that require two years. Unlike school-provided programs, hospital training leans heavily toward hands-on clinical work with less time in the classroom and additional reading and study at home. Training is also provided through the US Armed Forces.

It is important that prospective radiologic technologists attend an accredited program that will qualify for licensure. While it is not mandatory in all states, most hospitals and other employers strongly prefer graduates from accredited programs. It is not difficult to find an accredited program – there are nearly 1,000 of them in the US. The Joint Review Committee on Education in Radiologic Technology (JRCERT) accredits programs in radiography and the American Registry of Magnetic Resonance Imaging Technologists (ARMRIT) accredits MRI programs. You can find the schools with accredited programs nearest you by visiting the websites of these two organizations.

All training programs include both classroom study and clinical work. Classroom instruction typically covers:

- Anatomy and physiology
- Basic patient care
- Pathology
- Radiation physics and protection

- Image production and evaluation
- Medical terminology
- Equipment protocols
- Examination techniques
- Some schools also require medical coding and medical office courses.

Hands-on experience is a vital part of training. Students learn the techniques of the career in real clinical settings, observing at first before proceeding to work with actual patients. Before graduation, students will have learned how to operate equipment, properly position patients, how to follow safety protocols, acquire and calculate accurate mathematical measurements, organize and process medical images, and perform quality control.

There are two ways an individual can enter the field of radiologic technology with fewer than two years of training. There are certificate programs that last from six to 12 months available to experienced medical professionals in other health occupations, such as registered nurses, who want to change fields. Medical technologists or radiographers who have been on the job for a couple of years might also consider this kind of training in order to specialize in computerized tomography (CT), magnetic resonance imaging (MRI), or mammography.

For those who want to get started quickly and do not mind starting with a limited scope of practice, there are certificate programs for X-ray technicians that can take as few as six months to complete. X-ray technicians with this kind of training generally work in urgent care centers and doctor's offices, but not in hospitals.

Some colleges and universities offer a bachelor's degree in radiologic technology. Unlike many other healthcare professions, earning a four-year degree like this is not mandatory for most entry-level jobs. It is a good idea, however, for those wanting more in-depth study that could lead to more advancement opportunities in the future. A bachelor's or master's degree in one of the radiologic technologies is desirable for supervisory, administrative, or teaching positions.

Licensing and Certification

Most states require radiologic technologists to be licensed or certified. Even if a state does not require it, most employers expect prospective technologists to be certified.

Requirements for licensing vary by state. Typically, technologists need to graduate from an accredited program and pass a certification exam that is designed to adequately demonstrate knowledge and skills to enter the field. Some states conduct their own exams while others accept certification from a certifying body. Certifications for radiologic technologists are available from the American Registry of Radiologic Technologists (ARRT). This is the largest certification organization, with more than 300,000 professional radiologic technologists in its registry. MRI technologists can obtain certification from the ARRT or from the American Registry of Magnetic Resonance Imaging Technologists (ARMRIT).

EARNINGS

PERHAPS THE BEST REASON TO become a radiologic tech is the relatively high salary. The median annual wage for radiologic technologists is about $60,000. Considering it only takes two years to obtain the required education and training that is excellent. The top 10 percent do very well at $85,000 annually, while the lowest 10 percent earn almost $40,000.

Those who specialize in MRI technology do even better. The median annual wage for MRI technologists is about $70,000. The highest 10 percent earn more than $95,000 and the lowest 10 percent earn about $50,000.

As is the case with most professions, earnings vary depending on a number of factors, including geographic location, work experience, and education. Radiology techs can expect earnings to increase incrementally for each year on the job. Those with more than the minimum education often receive a higher starting pay and may be eligible for advancement opportunities with pay increases later on. These individuals are most likely to be top listed for future managerial positions, which typically offer a pay raise as well. With experience, additional education, or supervisory responsibilities, salaries can easily exceed $75,000 per year, depending on your area of specialization.

Compensation can vary somewhat among different industries employing radiologic technologists. For example, those who work in private medical practices do not do as well as those in medical and diagnostic laboratories. Surgical hospitals pay more than either of those, but the top paying employers are outpatient care centers where the average salary is $75,000, and specialty hospitals, such as cancer treatment centers.

Location makes a difference. Rurally based hospitals typically offer lower salaries than urban-based ones. The metropolitan areas where radiologic technologists earn the most are located in California and include Vallejo, San Jose, San Rafael, San Francisco, and Oakland. States with the highest salary for this profession include Massachusetts, Nevada, and Maryland.

Most radiologic technologists work full time. Because imaging is needed in emergency situations, some technologists work evenings, weekends, or on call. However, there is an upside to that. Many employers allow radiologic technologists to work flexible schedules, which provides time for family, school, or other activities. Full-time techs typically receive health insurance, sick leave, and retirement plans from their employers. Those working part time may not receive full benefits.

OPPORTUNITIES

THERE ARE APPROXIMATELY 215,000 radiology technologists in THE United States today, and the number of jobs in this field is expected to continue growing. Employment experts project employment of radiologic technologists to increase 12 percent over the next 10 years. That amounts to approximately 25,000 new jobs. The job outlook for certified MRI technologists is even better, with a projected growth rate of almost 15 percent over the same time period. This is a significantly faster growth rate than the average for all other occupations.

Imaging has become a routine diagnostic tool for most healthcare providers. Healthcare providers, large and small, need radiologic technologists to help doctors with diagnostic medical examinations. Job openings regularly occur when radiologic technologists retire, relocate, move into a new specialty, or advance into management.

The biggest contributor to job growth in this field is the large aging population, which is growing faster than the general population. As people age, there is usually an increase in medical conditions, such as cancer, Alzheimer's disease, arthritis, and bone fractures caused by osteoporosis. The demand is strong for radiologic technologists because imaging is needed to diagnose and treat these conditions.

To compete successfully for jobs, it is important to enroll only in accredited programs. The best job prospects are available to those who obtain multiple certifications. The ARRT offers certification in specialty areas including angiography, mammography, ultrasound, nuclear medicine, radiation therapy, MRI, or CT scanning. The most popular is MRI, the choice of more than half of all technologists looking to expand their options. It is a wise choice since job growth for MRI technologists is expected to be even better than for those in general radiology. It can also yield a salary increase of 25 percent or more.

Some radiologic technologists progress by becoming instructors with equipment manufacturers or vocational schools, while others take jobs as sales representatives.

Although the demand for radiologic technologists is strong across the board, not every city has the same level of opportunity. Radiologic technicians living in areas where there are fewer jobs should be flexible and willing to relocate to areas with more opportunities. This usually means moving from a small town to a larger city. Another way to deal with lack of opportunities is to become a traveling technologist. There are agencies that specifically connect technologists with jobs throughout the country. Traveling technologists are always needed to cover staff who may be on vacation, maternity or paternity leave, or are ill for an extended period of time.

Advancement Opportunities

Experienced radiologic technologists can move up the career ladder by advancing into a management role. The first step up would be shift supervisor, which involves supervising a team of radiologic technologists during their scheduled shifts. A successful shift supervisor can advance into the position of chief radiologic technologist. This usually requires a minimum of five years of experience and some employers require a college or business school degree. Ultimately, a technologist with the necessary educational background can move into the role of program director or department administrator. This usually requires a master's degree in business or health administration. Some institutions will accept the completion of certain courses in addition to proven managerial skills.

GETTING STARTED

START THE PROCESS OF FINDING YOUR FIRST JOB as a radiologic technologist while still in school. Get familiar with your school's career resource center. There you will find job postings and notices of upcoming job fairs. You can also get help with writing résumés and pick up some interview tips.

Networking is the most productive method of finding jobs and advancing in healthcare careers.

Your professors will be your first contacts. It is common for instructors to be either currently active in the field or retired with an extensive background as a working professional. Either way, they can point you in the right direction to start your job search.

Continue doing everything you can to make networking contacts. Some of your most valuable contacts will be made through internships and volunteer positions. In addition to networking opportunities, these kinds of on-the-job training provide an excellent way to obtain real-world experience and learn the relevant medical lingo. For volunteer opportunities, go to the nearest hospital and offer to help out in the imaging department. For best results, go directly to the department head with your offer.

Internships can put you in contact with potential employers. As an intern, you will receive first-hand knowledge of the daily routines while preparing yourself for a possible transition into a full-time position. Depending on your education track, an internship may be required to qualify for graduation. In that case, your school will help you find an internship program. You can also locate your own internship through hospitals and other healthcare providers.

Join professional associations such as the American Society of Radiologic Technologists (ASRT). Not only do these organizations offer plenty of networking opportunities, but they also post open positions on their websites. Make the most of your membership by participating in workshops, seminars, and other events. It is a good way to stay current on trends and connect with leaders in the radiologic sciences.

Your first job does not need to be the result of a referral. You can submit "cold" applications directly to hospitals, doctors, dentists, and imaging labs. Online job boards, especially those dedicated to the healthcare field, are an excellent source of job leads. There may be tons of openings, but be sure to personalize each and every cover letter for best results. Also, look for healthcare-related job placement agencies. These agencies are well connected to hospitals all around the country and can help you find jobs you might not have found on your own. Some specialize in placing traveling technologists in temporary positions that typically last two or three months. If you want to see the country, this is a great way to explore the many career paths that may be open to you.

Take advantage of opportunities to learn new skills and try new things. Being flexible is very appealing to potential employers. Be willing to perform different tasks and look for opportunities to cross-train. You can get a significant leg up in finding employment by getting additional certifications.

ASSOCIATIONS

■ **American Society of Radiologic Technologists (ASRT)**
www.asrt.org

■ **American Registry of Radiologic Technologists (ARRT)**
www.arrt.org

■ **Joint Review Committee on Education in Radiologic Technology**
www.jrcert.org

■ **American Registry of Magnetic Resonance Imaging Technologists**
www.armrit.org

■ **American Association of Medical Dosimetrists**
www.medicaldosimetry.org

PERIODICALS

■ **Radiologic Technology**
www.radiologictechnology.org

■ **Radiology Today**
www.radiologytoday.net

■ **Applied Radiology**
www.appliedradiology.com

www.ingramcontent.com/pod-product-compliance
Lightning Source LLC
Chambersburg PA
CBHW071200220526
45468CB00003B/1103